How to Have Amazing Sex

Introduction: Setting the Stage for Incredible Intimacy

Welcome to "How to Have Amazing Sex" – an immersive journey into the intricate realms of intimacy, pleasure, and profound connection. Within these pages, we're embarking on a transformative exploration that transcends mere physical gratification and delves into the depths of human desire and fulfillment.

Sexuality, as we understand it, is a multifaceted aspect of our existence, intricately woven into the fabric of our identities, relationships, and experiences. Yet, despite its profound significance, it often remains shrouded in secrecy, misinformation, and societal taboos. This book seeks to peel back those layers of uncertainty and shine a light on the beauty and complexity of sexual expression.

Our journey begins with a fundamental question: What is "amazing sex"? While the term may conjure images of wild passion and intense physical pleasure, its essence extends far beyond mere moments of ecstasy. Amazing sex encompasses a holistic experience that intertwines the physical, emotional, and spiritual aspects of intimacy. It's about forging deep connections with ourselves and our partners, exploring our desires with curiosity and openness, and embracing vulnerability as a gateway to profound connection.

Throughout these pages, we'll navigate the intricate terrain of human sexuality, starting with a thorough exploration of our bodies and desires. Understanding ourselves—our anatomy, our preferences, our boundaries—is essential for cultivating fulfilling sexual experiences. We'll delve into the intricacies of pleasure, exploring the myriad ways in which our bodies respond to stimulation and discovering new pathways to ecstasy.

But amazing sex isn't just about the physical act—it's also about communication, trust, and mutual understanding. We'll delve into the importance of open and honest dialogue about our desires, fears, and boundaries, creating a foundation of trust and intimacy that enhances our sexual encounters.

As we journey deeper into the realms of sexual exploration, we'll uncover the power of fantasy, role-play, and experimentation, embracing the full spectrum of human desire and imagination. We'll learn how to unleash our inhibitions, let go of societal norms, and embrace the wild, untamed aspects of our sexuality.

Yet, our exploration doesn't end between the sheets. We'll also address the challenges and obstacles that may arise on our journey, from physical issues like erectile dysfunction or pain during intercourse to emotional barriers stemming from past trauma or societal stigma. With empathy and understanding, we'll navigate these challenges together, offering practical advice and support to help you overcome any obstacles standing in the way of truly amazing sex.

Ultimately, the path to amazing sex is a deeply personal one, shaped by our unique experiences, desires, and aspirations. Whether you're embarking on a journey of self-discovery, seeking to reignite the flames of passion in a long-term relationship, or simply curious to explore new realms of pleasure, this book is your guide.

So let's embark on this journey together—a journey of self-discovery, intimacy, and unparalleled pleasure. Let's unlock the secrets to truly amazing sex and embrace the full potential of our sexual selves.

Understanding Your Body: Embracing Self-Awareness and Sexual Exploration

the intricate tapestry of human sexuality, one of the most profound and empowering journeys begins with a deep understanding of one's own body. This chapter serves as a comprehensive guide, viting you to embark on a voyage of self-discovery where curiosity meets exploration and self-awareness blossoms into empowerment.

Anatomy: Mapping the Terrain of Pleasure

nderstanding the anatomy of pleasure is the first step towards unlocking its secrets. From the :ternal erogenous zones like the lips, nipples, and genitals, to the internal structures such as the itoris, G-spot, and prostate, delving into the intricate landscape of human anatomy offers a >admap to heightened pleasure. By familiarizing yourself with the physical structures and echanisms involved in arousal and orgasm, you gain insight into the pathways to ecstasy that lie ithin your own body.

Pleasure Mapping: Charting Your Erotic Landscape

easure mapping is a deeply personal journey of self-exploration, where you become the rtographer of your own erotic landscape. Through experimentation and introspection, you identify id explore your individual pleasure points, uncovering the unique patterns and preferences that ing you the most satisfaction. Whether through solo exploration or with the guidance of a trusted artner, this process of discovery is a celebration of self-awareness and empowerment.

Mind-Body Connection: Cultivating Sensual Awareness

t the heart of sexual exploration lies the profound connection between mind and body. Cultivating :nsual awareness involves tuning into the subtle nuances of physical sensation, embracing indfulness practices, and engaging in sensory exercises that heighten your awareness of pleasure. / learning to listen to your body's signals and cues, you deepen your capacity for presence and ijoyment during sexual experiences, fostering a deeper sense of intimacy and connection.

Sexual Response Cycle: Navigating the Peaks and Valleys

nderstanding the intricacies of the sexual response cycle is essential for navigating the peaks and illeys of arousal and pleasure. From the initial spark of desire to the crescendo of orgasm and the :ntle descent back to a state of relaxation, each phase of the sexual response cycle offers its own ique pleasures and challenges. By recognizing the dynamic nature of sexual response and honoring the rhythms of your own body, you cultivate a deeper appreciation for the complexity of sexual experience.

5. Exploring Sensation: From Sensory Play to Erotic Experimentation

Sensation is the currency of erotic exploration, offering an infinite array of possibilities for pleasure and connection. From the gentle caress of a lover's hand to the exhilarating intensity of a spanking or nipple stimulation, exploring sensation involves embracing the full spectrum of tactile, auditory, olfactory, and gustatory experiences. By experimenting with different textures, temperatures, pressures, and sensations, you expand your erotic repertoire and deepen your connection to pleasure.

6. Body Image and Self-Acceptance: Embracing Your Erotic Self

Body image and self-acceptance are integral aspects of sexual empowerment, challenging societal norms and expectations surrounding beauty and desirability. Embracing your erotic self involves cultivating a sense of self-compassion and acceptance, recognizing the inherent beauty and uniqueness of your own body. By celebrating your body as a source of pleasure and joy, you reclaim agency over your own sexual narrative, embracing authenticity and vulnerability as pathways to true intimacy and connection.

In essence, understanding your body is not just a journey of physical exploration, but a profound voyage of self-discovery and empowerment. By embracing self-awareness and delving into the depths of your own erotic landscape, you lay the foundation for a lifetime of pleasure, connection, and fulfillment. So, let us embark on this journey together, honoring the wisdom of our bodies and reveling in the infinite possibilities of sexual exploration.

Communication is Key: Navigating Open and Honest Dialogue About Sex

In the realm of human sexuality, communication serves as the cornerstone upon which fulfilling and enriching experiences are built. This chapter delves into the crucial role of communication in sexual intimacy, guiding you through the process of fostering open and honest dialogue with your partner(s) about desires, boundaries, and fantasies.

1. The Importance of Communication in Sexuality

Communication is the lifeblood of sexual connection, providing a pathway for understanding, empathy, and mutual satisfaction. By engaging in open and honest dialogue about your desires, fears, and boundaries, you create a foundation of trust and intimacy that enhances the quality of your sexual experiences. Recognizing the power of communication to deepen connection and foster intimacy is the first step towards cultivating a fulfilling and satisfying sex life.

2. Creating a Safe Space for Dialogue

Building a safe space for sexual communication involves creating an environment of trust, respect, and non-judgment where both partners feel comfortable expressing their desires and concerns. Establishing ground rules for communication, such as active listening, empathy, and honesty, helps to foster a sense of mutual respect and understanding. By prioritizing emotional safety and vulnerability, you create the conditions for authentic and meaningful dialogue about sex.

3. Initiating Difficult Conversations

Navigating difficult conversations about sex requires courage, empathy, and vulnerability. Whether addressing concerns about sexual performance, exploring new fantasies, or discussing past traumas, approaching these topics with sensitivity and compassion is essential. By communicating your needs and desires with clarity and honesty, you pave the way for deeper connection and understanding with your partner(s).

4. Active Listening and Empathy

Active listening and empathy are essential skills for effective sexual communication. By tuning into your partner's verbal and nonverbal cues, you demonstrate respect and validation for their experiences and feelings. Cultivating empathy allows you to understand your partner's perspective and respond with sensitivity and compassion, fostering a deeper sense of connection and intimacy in your relationship.

5. Expressing Desires and Boundaries

Expressing your desires and boundaries openly and honestly is essential for creating mutual satisfaction and fulfillment in sexual encounters. Whether it's communicating your preferences for specific activities, discussing boundaries around consent and safety, or expressing fantasies and desires, being clear and direct in your communication ensures that both partners feel respected and valued. By honoring each other's boundaries and desires, you create a space where trust and intimacy can flourish.

6. Negotiating Consent

Negotiating consent is a fundamental aspect of sexual communication, ensuring that all parties involved feel safe, respected, and empowered. Consent is an ongoing process that involves active communication, mutual agreement, and respect for each other's boundaries. By seeking enthusiastic consent and respecting verbal and nonverbal cues, you create a culture of consent that promotes mutual respect and autonomy in sexual encounters.

In essence, communication is the foundation upon which fulfilling and satisfying sexual experiences are built. By fostering open and honest dialogue about desires, boundaries, and fantasies, you create a space where trust, intimacy, and mutual satisfaction can thrive. So, let us embark on this journey together, honoring the power of communication to deepen connection and enrich our sexual experiences.

The Art of Foreplay: Building Anticipation and Enhancing Pleasure

Foreplay is often regarded as the gateway to truly fulfilling and satisfying sexual experiences. In this chapter, we'll explore the intricacies of foreplay, delving into the myriad ways in which it can build anticipation, heighten arousal, and amplify pleasure for both partners.

1. Understanding Foreplay: Beyond a Prelude to Sex

Foreplay is not merely a prelude to intercourse; it's an essential component of sexual intimacy in its own right. By shifting our perspective to view foreplay as an integral part of the sexual experience, we can unlock its full potential to enhance pleasure and deepen connection.

2. The Power of Anticipation: Building Sexual Tension

Anticipation is a potent aphrodisiac, fueling desire and heightening arousal. Through teasing glances, whispered promises, and playful touches, you can build sexual tension and anticipation, creating a sense of longing and excitement that intensifies the pleasure of the eventual release.

3. Sensual Touch: Exploring Erogenous Zones

Sensual touch is the cornerstone of foreplay, offering a rich tapestry of sensations that ignite desire and pleasure. By exploring each other's erogenous zones—from the lips and neck to the breasts, nipples, and genitals—you can discover new pathways to arousal and ecstasy, deepening your connection with your partner(s) and amplifying the intensity of your sexual experiences.

4. Verbal Foreplay: Erotic Communication and Dirty Talk

Verbal foreplay encompasses a wide range of erotic communication, from whispered confessions of desire to explicit descriptions of fantasies and desires. By engaging in dirty talk and erotic storytelling, you can heighten anticipation, stimulate the imagination, and ignite passion, creating a rich tapestry of words that enhances the pleasure of physical touch.

5. Nonverbal Communication: The Language of Desire

Nonverbal communication plays a crucial role in foreplay, allowing partners to express desire, arousal, and pleasure through gestures, body language, and facial expressions. By tuning into your partner's nonverbal cues and responding with sensitivity and attentiveness, you can deepen your connection and synchronize your movements in a dance of desire and passion.

6. Creative Exploration: Experimenting with New Techniques and Activities

Foreplay offers endless opportunities for creative exploration and experimentation. From sensual massage and playful tickling to erotic games and role-play scenarios, you can explore a diverse array of techniques and activities that cater to your individual desires and fantasies, enriching your sexual repertoire and deepening your connection with your partner(s).

7. Extended Foreplay: Savoring the Journey

In the rush towards orgasm, it's easy to overlook the pleasure of the journey itself. Extended foreplay allows you to savor each moment, indulging in the pleasure of anticipation and exploration without the pressure of reaching a predetermined destination. By slowing down and focusing on the sensations of the present moment, you can heighten arousal, intensify pleasure, and deepen intimacy with your partner(s).

In essence, foreplay is an art form—a delicate dance of anticipation, exploration, and connection that lays the foundation for truly fulfilling and satisfying sexual experiences. By embracing the power of anticipation, exploring each other's bodies and desires, and savoring the journey of pleasure, you can elevate your sexual encounters to new heights of intimacy and ecstasy. So, let us embark on this journey together, honoring the art of foreplay as a pathway to profound pleasure and connection.

Exploring Sexual Fantasies and Desires: Embracing Variety and Adventure

Human sexuality is a vast and endlessly diverse landscape, filled with an infinite array of fantasies, desires, and possibilities. In this chapter, we'll embark on a journey of exploration and discovery, delving into the rich tapestry of sexual fantasies and desires, and embracing the exhilarating adventure of sexual exploration.

The Role of Sexual Fantasies: Unleashing the Power of Imagination

Sexual fantasies serve as windows into the deepest recesses of our desires and imaginations. They allow us to explore taboo desires, fulfill unmet needs, and indulge in flights of erotic fancy that transcend the constraints of reality. By embracing our fantasies with curiosity and openness, we can unlock their transformative power to enhance pleasure and deepen intimacy.

Understanding Fantasy Dynamics: Taboo, Role-Play, and Beyond

Sexual fantasies come in many shapes and forms, ranging from the taboo and forbidden to the playful and adventurous. Whether exploring power dynamics, engaging in role-play scenarios, or indulging in fetishistic desires, understanding the dynamics of fantasy allows us to navigate their complexities with creativity and consent, fostering a sense of exploration and discovery in our sexual encounters.

Communicating Fantasies with Your Partner(s): Building Trust and Connection

Sharing our sexual fantasies with a partner requires courage, vulnerability, and trust. By initiating open and honest conversations about our desires and boundaries, we create a safe space for mutual exploration and expression, deepening our connection and intimacy with our partner(s) in the process. Whether through whispered confessions, erotic storytelling, or shared fantasies, communicating our desires allows us to embark on a collaborative journey of sexual exploration and fulfillment.

Experimenting with Fantasy Fulfillment: From Simulation to Reality

Fantasy fulfillment offers endless opportunities for exploration and adventure. Whether enacting role-play scenarios, exploring BDSM dynamics, or experimenting with erotic accessories and toys, embracing our fantasies in the bedroom allows us to transform our deepest desires into tangible experiences of pleasure and fulfillment. By stepping outside our comfort zones and embracing the unknown, we open ourselves up to new realms of excitement and discovery in our sexual encounters.

5. Navigating Boundaries and Consent: Respecting Limits and Honoring Autonomy

While exploring sexual fantasies can be exhilarating and liberating, it's essential to navigate boundaries and consent with care and respect. Honoring our own limits and those of our partner(s) ensures that all parties feel safe, respected, and empowered in their sexual experiences. By prioritizing clear communication, enthusiastic consent, and mutual respect, we create a foundation of trust and safety that allows us to explore our fantasies with confidence and joy.

6. Fantasy Exploration as a Lifelong Journey: Embracing Evolution and Growth

Our sexual fantasies are not static; they evolve and change over time in response to our experiences, desires, and relationships. Embracing the journey of fantasy exploration as a lifelong adventure allows us to continually discover new facets of ourselves and our desires, deepening our connection with our own sexuality and enhancing the richness of our intimate relationships. By remaining open to growth, evolution, and transformation, we can embrace the infinite possibilities of sexual exploration with a sense of curiosity, wonder, and joy.

In essence, exploring sexual fantasies and desires is a deeply personal and profoundly liberating journey—a journey of self-discovery, adventure, and fulfillment. By embracing the power of imagination, communicating openly with our partner(s), and navigating boundaries with care and respect, we can unlock the transformative potential of fantasy exploration and embark on a lifelong odyssey of sexual discovery and fulfillment. So, let us embark on this journey together, embracing the exhilarating adventure of sexual exploration with curiosity, courage, and joy.

Mastering Techniques: From Kissing to Orgasm, Tips for Mind-Blowing Sex

Sexual mastery is not just about technique; it's about understanding the nuances of pleasure, communication, and connection. In this chapter, we'll explore a range of techniques designed to elevate your sexual experiences to new heights of ecstasy and satisfaction.

1. The Art of Kissing: Igniting Passion and Connection

Kissing is the gateway to intimacy, a sensual dance of lips and tongues that ignites passion and deepens connection. By exploring different techniques—from gentle pecks to passionate lip locks—you can unlock the transformative power of kissing, infusing your encounters with an electrifying spark of desire and arousal.

2. Foreplay Techniques: Building Anticipation and Heightening Pleasure

Foreplay is a playground of sensory delights, offering endless opportunities for exploration and arousal. From sensual massages and tantalizing caresses to playful teasing and erotic nibbling, mastering the art of foreplay allows you to build anticipation, heighten arousal, and create a foundation of pleasure that sets the stage for mind-blowing sex.

3. Oral Pleasure: Giving and Receiving with Skill and Enthusiasm

Oral sex is a deeply intimate and intensely pleasurable experience that can bring both partners to the heights of ecstasy. Whether giving or receiving, mastering the art of oral pleasure involves techniques such as varying pressure and speed, exploring different angles and rhythms, and paying close attention to your partner's responses and cues. By approaching oral sex with skill, enthusiasm, and a spirit of exploration, you can unlock new dimensions of pleasure and intimacy in your sexual encounters.

4. Penetrative Techniques: Maximizing Pleasure and Connection

Penetrative sex offers a profound opportunity for connection and pleasure, but it's not just about thrusting; it's about rhythm, depth, and angle. By exploring different positions, angles, and movements, you can maximize pleasure for both partners and deepen your connection in the process. From slow and sensual lovemaking to passionate and intense thrusting, mastering penetrative techniques allows you to tailor your sexual encounters to suit your desires and preferences.

5. Orgasmic Techniques: Unlocking the Keys to Climax

Orgasm is the pinnacle of sexual pleasure, a transcendent moment of release and ecstasy that leaves both partners feeling deeply fulfilled and satisfied. By exploring techniques such as edging, breath control, and kegel exercises, you can enhance your ability to experience and prolong orgasm, unlocking new levels of pleasure and intensity in your sexual encounters. By mastering the art of orgasmic techniques, you can cultivate a deeper connection with your own body and unleash its full potential for pleasure and satisfaction.

6. Aftercare: Nurturing Connection and Intimacy

Aftercare is an essential part of sexual mastery, offering a space for connection, reassurance, and emotional bonding after intense sexual experiences. Whether cuddling, kissing, or engaging in quiet conversation, taking the time to nurture each other's emotional and physical well-being fosters a deeper sense of intimacy and connection, ensuring that your sexual encounters leave both partners feeling cherished, supported, and deeply satisfied.

In essence, mastering sexual techniques is about more than just physical skill; it's about understanding the nuances of pleasure, communication, and connection. By exploring a range of techniques—from kissing and foreplay to oral sex, penetrative techniques, and orgasmic techniques—you can elevate your sexual experiences to new heights of ecstasy and satisfaction. So, let us embark on this journey together, embracing the art of sexual mastery with curiosity, enthusiasm, and a spirit of exploration.

Overcoming Challenges: Addressing Common Issues and Enhancing Intimacy

Sexual intimacy, like any aspect of human connection, is not immune to challenges. In this chapter, we'll explore common issues that couples may face in their sexual relationships and provide strategies for overcoming these obstacles, fostering deeper intimacy and satisfaction in the process.

1. Communication Breakdown: Restoring Dialogue and Trust

Communication breakdowns can hinder sexual intimacy, leading to misunderstandings, frustrations, and feelings of disconnect. By prioritizing open and honest communication, couples can address underlying issues, express their needs and desires, and rebuild trust and connection in their sexual relationship. Techniques such as active listening, empathy, and validation can help couples navigate difficult conversations and strengthen their bond.

2. Performance Anxiety: Managing Pressure and Expectations

Performance anxiety is a common issue that can impact sexual satisfaction and enjoyment. By reframing sex as a collaborative and exploratory experience rather than a performance, couples can alleviate pressure and expectations, allowing for greater relaxation and enjoyment. Techniques such as mindfulness, deep breathing, and sensate focus exercises can help individuals overcome performance anxiety and reconnect with their bodies and desires.

3. Desire Discrepancy: Bridging the Gap

Desire discrepancy occurs when partners have differing levels of sexual desire, leading to feelings of frustration, rejection, and resentment. By acknowledging and validating each other's desires, couples can work together to bridge the gap and find creative solutions that meet both partners' needs. Techniques such as scheduling intimacy, exploring new activities, and prioritizing non-sexual forms of connection can help couples navigate desire differences and cultivate a more satisfying sexual relationship.

4. Body Image Issues: Cultivating Self-Acceptance and Empathy

Body image issues can undermine sexual confidence and enjoyment, leading to feelings of insecurity and self-consciousness. By fostering self-acceptance and compassion, individuals can overcome negative body image and embrace their bodies as sources of pleasure and joy. Techniques such as self-affirmations, body-positive practices, and sensual self-care rituals can help individuals cultivate a more positive relationship with their bodies and enhance sexual intimacy.

5. Past Trauma: Healing Wounds and Reclaiming Pleasure

Past trauma, whether physical or emotional, can profoundly impact sexual intimacy, leading to feelings of fear, shame, and disconnection. By seeking support from qualified professionals, individuals can address past trauma and reclaim agency over their bodies and desires. Techniques such as trauma-informed therapy, mindfulness practices, and gradual exposure exercises can help individuals heal from past wounds and cultivate a sense of safety and empowerment in their sexual relationships.

6. Relationship Dynamics: Navigating Power and Control

Relationship dynamics such as unequal power dynamics or issues of control can disrupt sexual intimacy, leading to feelings of resentment, frustration, and disconnection. By fostering equality and mutual respect in their relationship, couples can create a foundation of trust and safety that enhances sexual intimacy. Techniques such as setting boundaries, negotiating consent, and engaging in collaborative decision-making can help couples navigate power dynamics and cultivate a more fulfilling and satisfying sexual relationship.

In essence, overcoming challenges in sexual intimacy requires a combination of compassion, communication, and collaboration. By addressing common issues such as communication breakdowns, performance anxiety, desire discrepancy, body image issues, past trauma, and relationship dynamics, couples can deepen their connection and enhance their sexual satisfaction. So, let us embark on this journey together, embracing the opportunity to overcome challenges and foster deeper intimacy and connection in our sexual relationships.

he Role of Emotional Connection: Cultivating Intimacy Beyond the Physical

n the realm of human sexuality, emotional connection serves as the bedrock upon which profound ntimacy and fulfillment are built. This chapter explores the pivotal role of emotional connection in exual relationships, offering insights and strategies for cultivating deeper intimacy beyond the hysical realm.

. Understanding Emotional Connection: The Heartbeat of Intimacy

motional connection is the essence of true intimacy, encompassing trust, vulnerability, and mutual nderstanding between partners. It goes beyond physical attraction and sexual chemistry, fostering sense of closeness and belonging that nourishes the soul. By recognizing the importance of motional connection, couples can lay the foundation for a deeply fulfilling and satisfying sexual elationship.

. Building Trust and Vulnerability: The Pillars of Emotional Intimacy

rust and vulnerability are the cornerstones of emotional intimacy, creating a safe space where artners feel seen, heard, and accepted for who they truly are. By sharing their fears, hopes, and reams with each other, couples deepen their connection and strengthen their bond. Techniques uch as active listening, empathy, and validation can help couples cultivate trust and vulnerability in heir relationship, fostering a deeper sense of emotional intimacy.

. Communicating Emotions: The Language of the Heart

ffective communication is essential for nurturing emotional connection, allowing partners to xpress their feelings, needs, and desires with honesty and clarity. By practicing open and honest ommunication, couples can deepen their understanding of each other and strengthen their motional bond. Techniques such as reflective listening, expressing gratitude, and using "I" tatements can help couples communicate their emotions in a way that fosters connection and ntimacy.

. Nurturing Affection and Intimacy: Gestures of Love and Care

ffection and intimacy are expressed not only through words but also through actions. Simple estures of love and care—such as holding hands, cuddling, or sharing a heartfelt embrace—can trengthen the emotional connection between partners and deepen their sense of intimacy. By prioritizing physical touch and affection in their relationship, couples can create moments of connection and closeness that enhance their emotional bond.

5. Sharing Values and Goals: Creating a Shared Vision for the Future

Shared values and goals provide a sense of purpose and direction in a relationship, fostering a sense of unity and cohesion between partners. By discussing their hopes, dreams, and aspirations with each other, couples can create a shared vision for the future and strengthen their emotional connection. Techniques such as goal-setting, brainstorming, and vision boarding can help couples align their values and goals, fostering a sense of partnership and collaboration in their relationship.

6. Resolving Conflict and Reconnecting: The Path to Deeper Understanding

Conflict is a natural part of any relationship, but how couples navigate conflict can either deepen or erode their emotional connection. By approaching conflict with empathy, understanding, and a willingness to compromise, couples can resolve disagreements in a way that strengthens their emotional bond. Techniques such as active listening, de-escalation strategies, and collaborative problem-solving can help couples reconnect and reaffirm their commitment to each other.

In essence, emotional connection is the heart and soul of sexual intimacy, infusing relationships with warmth, depth, and meaning. By prioritizing trust, vulnerability, communication, affection, shared values, and conflict resolution, couples can cultivate a deeper sense of emotional connection that enriches their sexual relationship and fosters lasting intimacy and fulfillment. So, let us embark on this journey together, embracing the transformative power of emotional connection in our sexual relationships.

Safer Sex Practices: Protecting Your Health and Well-Being

Sexual health and well-being are paramount in any intimate relationship. This chapter explores essential safer sex practices that prioritize the health and safety of all partners, empowering individuals to enjoy fulfilling and responsible sexual experiences.

1. Understanding Safer Sex: Prioritizing Health and Safety

Safer sex encompasses a range of practices aimed at reducing the risk of sexually transmitted infections (STIs) and unwanted pregnancies. By prioritizing health and safety, individuals can engage in sexual encounters with confidence and peace of mind, knowing that they are taking proactive steps to protect themselves and their partners.

2. Condom Use: Barrier Protection for STI Prevention

Condoms are one of the most effective methods for preventing the transmission of STIs and reducing the risk of unintended pregnancies. By using condoms consistently and correctly during vaginal, anal, and oral sex, individuals can significantly reduce their risk of contracting or spreading STIs, including HIV, gonorrhea, chlamydia, and herpes.

3. Regular Testing: Knowledge is Power

Regular testing for STIs is essential for maintaining sexual health and well-being. By getting tested regularly and encouraging their partners to do the same, individuals can detect and treat STIs early, reducing the risk of complications and transmission to others. Testing for STIs such as HIV, syphilis, gonorrhea, chlamydia, and HPV should be a routine part of sexual health maintenance.

4. Communication About STIs: Honest and Open Dialogue

Open and honest communication about STIs is crucial for promoting safer sex practices and reducing the risk of transmission. By discussing STI status, testing history, and safer sex practices with their partners, individuals can make informed decisions about their sexual health and well-being. Creating a safe space for dialogue eliminates stigma and fosters trust and transparency in intimate relationships.

5. PrEP and PEP: Additional Tools for HIV Prevention

Pre-exposure prophylaxis (PrEP) and post-exposure prophylaxis (PEP) are additional tools for preventing HIV transmission in high-risk individuals. PrEP involves taking a daily medication to reduce the risk of HIV acquisition, while PEP involves taking medication after potential exposure to HIV to prevent infection. Individuals at increased risk of HIV transmission, such as those with HIV-positive partners or individuals engaging in high-risk sexual behaviors, may benefit from PrEP or PEP.

6. Consent and Boundaries: Essential Components of Safer Sex

Consent and boundaries are foundational principles of safer sex practices, ensuring that all sexual encounters are consensual and respectful. By obtaining enthusiastic consent and respecting each other's boundaries, individuals can create a safe and empowering sexual environment that prioritizes mutual respect and autonomy. Consensual sex is not only ethically responsible but also essential for promoting positive sexual experiences and healthy relationships.

In essence, safer sex practices are essential for protecting the health and well-being of all partners and promoting positive sexual experiences. By prioritizing barrier protection, regular testing, open communication, and informed decision-making, individuals can enjoy fulfilling and responsible sexual encounters while minimizing the risk of STIs and unwanted pregnancies. So, let us embark on this journey together, embracing the importance of safer sex practices in promoting sexual health and well-being for all.

Beyond the Bedroom: Integrating Sexuality into Daily Life and Relationships

Sexuality is not confined to the bedroom; it permeates every aspect of our lives and relationships. This chapter explores the ways in which individuals can embrace and integrate their sexuality into their daily lives and relationships, fostering deeper connection, fulfillment, and authenticity.

1. Embracing Sensuality: Cultivating Awareness and Presence

Sensuality is a mindset—a way of engaging with the world that embraces pleasure, beauty, and connection. By cultivating awareness and presence in everyday experiences, individuals can tap into their innate sensuality and infuse their lives with moments of joy, pleasure, and connection. Techniques such as mindfulness, sensory exploration, and conscious breathing can help individuals embrace their sensuality and live more fully in the present moment.

2. Eroticizing Everyday Activities: Finding Pleasure in the Ordinary

Eroticizing everyday activities involves infusing mundane tasks with a sense of playfulness, creativity, and sensuality. By approaching tasks such as cooking, cleaning, or gardening with a spirit of exploration and curiosity, individuals can discover new sources of pleasure and connection in their daily lives. Techniques such as mindful eating, sensory awareness, and playful experimentation can help individuals find pleasure in the ordinary and embrace the erotic potential of everyday experiences.

3. Flirting and Playfulness: Keeping the Spark Alive

Flirting and playfulness are essential ingredients for maintaining passion and connection in a relationship. By engaging in playful banter, spontaneous gestures, and flirtatious encounters, individuals can keep the spark alive and inject excitement into their relationship. Techniques such as playful teasing, surprise gifts, and shared adventures can help couples reconnect and rediscover the joy of playful intimacy.

4. Erotic Communication: Cultivating Intimate Connection

Erotic communication goes beyond words; it involves expressing desire, passion, and vulnerability in both verbal and nonverbal ways. By engaging in erotic communication with their partners, individuals can deepen their intimate connection and foster a sense of closeness and understanding. Techniques such as sexting, erotic storytelling, and sensual touch can help couples cultivate a rich and fulfilling erotic connection outside the bedroom.

5. Prioritizing Intimacy: Making Time for Connection

Intimacy requires time and attention, and it's essential to prioritize connection in daily life. By carving out dedicated time for intimacy and connection—whether through date nights, shared hobbies, or meaningful conversations—couples can strengthen their bond and deepen their emotional and sexual connection. Techniques such as scheduling regular check-ins, planning romantic getaways, and practicing active listening can help couples prioritize intimacy and connection in their relationship.

6. Self-Care and Self-Exploration: Nurturing Sexual Well-Being

Self-care and self-exploration are essential components of sexual well-being, allowing individuals to nurture their own needs, desires, and pleasures. By prioritizing self-care practices such as exercise, meditation, and creative expression, individuals can cultivate a sense of vitality and aliveness that enriches their sexual experiences. Techniques such as solo exploration, fantasy exploration, and self-pleasure rituals can help individuals deepen their connection with their own bodies and desires, fostering a sense of empowerment and self-love.

In essence, integrating sexuality into daily life and relationships is about embracing pleasure, connection, and authenticity in every moment. By cultivating sensuality, eroticizing everyday activities, embracing playfulness and flirtation, prioritizing intimacy, and nurturing sexual well-being, individuals can create a life filled with joy, passion, and fulfillment. So, let us embark on this journey together, embracing the beauty and richness of integrating sexuality into every aspect of our lives and relationships.

Maintaining Passion: Nurturing Long-Term Sexual Fulfillment

Sustaining passion in a long-term relationship requires dedication, creativity, and a commitment to ongoing growth and exploration. In this chapter, we'll explore strategies for nurturing passion and cultivating long-term sexual fulfillment, allowing couples to continue to deepen their connection and enjoyment over time.

. Prioritizing Connection: Cultivating Emotional Intimacy

Emotional intimacy is the foundation of sexual passion in a long-term relationship. By prioritizing open communication, empathy, and vulnerability, couples can deepen their emotional connection and strengthen their bond. Regular check-ins, shared experiences, and quality time together can help couples cultivate emotional intimacy and lay the groundwork for sustained passion.

. Keeping Things Fresh: Embracing Novelty and Variety

Novelty and variety are essential ingredients for maintaining passion in a long-term relationship. By exploring new activities, trying new experiences, and introducing novelty into their routine, couples can keep things exciting and spark new levels of desire and arousal. Date nights, weekend getaways, and trying new hobbies together can help couples infuse their relationship with freshness and excitement.

. Exploring Fantasies and Desires: Fostering Erotic Discovery

Exploring fantasies and desires allows couples to tap into their deepest desires and fantasies, creating opportunities for erotic discovery and adventure. By sharing fantasies, trying new activities, and exploring each other's desires with curiosity and openness, couples can keep the flame of passion alive and ignite new levels of excitement in their sexual relationship. Role-play, fantasy sharing, and experimenting with new techniques or toys can help couples explore their erotic potential and deepen their connection.

. Maintaining Physical Intimacy: Prioritizing Touch and Affection

Physical intimacy is essential for maintaining passion in a long-term relationship. By prioritizing touch, affection, and sensual connection, couples can keep the spark alive and deepen their physical bond. Regular physical affection, spontaneous gestures of love, and prioritizing cuddling and kissing can help couples maintain physical intimacy and sustain passion over time.

5. Communicating Needs and Desires: Honoring Individual and Shared Pleasures

Open communication about needs and desires is crucial for maintaining passion in a long-term relationship. By expressing their desires and preferences with honesty and vulnerability, couples can create a shared understanding of each other's needs and desires, fostering a deeper connection and enhancing sexual satisfaction. Regular check-ins, honest conversations, and mutual exploration can help couples navigate changes in desire and ensure that both partners feel valued and fulfilled.

6. Cultivating Gratitude and Appreciation: Nourishing Love and Connection

Cultivating gratitude and appreciation for each other is essential for sustaining passion in a long-term relationship. By expressing appreciation for their partner's qualities, gestures, and efforts, couples can nurture love and connection and strengthen their bond. Regular expressions of gratitude, acts of kindness, and acknowledging each other's contributions can help couples maintain a sense of closeness and intimacy and sustain passion over time.

In essence, maintaining passion in a long-term relationship requires dedication, effort, and a commitment to ongoing growth and exploration. By prioritizing connection, embracing novelty and variety, exploring fantasies and desires, maintaining physical intimacy, communicating needs and desires, and cultivating gratitude and appreciation, couples can nurture long-term sexual fulfillment and continue to deepen their connection and enjoyment over time. So, let us embark on this journey together, embracing the beauty and richness of sustaining passion in a long-term relationship.

Conclusion: Embracing Your Sexual Journey and Celebrating Amazing Sex

Congratulations! You've embarked on a journey of self-discovery, exploration, and growth—a journey that has taken you through the depths of desire, the heights of pleasure, and the complexities of intimacy. Along the way, you've learned valuable insights, discovered new techniques, and cultivated deeper connections with yourself and your partner(s).

As you reflect on your sexual journey, remember that it is a deeply personal and profoundly empowering experience—one that is uniquely yours to explore and embrace. Whether you're single or in a committed relationship, whether you're exploring new horizons or deepening existing connections, your sexuality is an integral part of who you are—a source of pleasure, fulfillment, and joy.

Throughout this book, you've discovered the importance of communication, the power of exploration, and the transformative potential of intimacy. You've learned to prioritize your needs and desires, to embrace vulnerability and authenticity, and to celebrate the beauty and diversity of human sexuality.

As you continue on your journey, remember to be gentle with yourself, to practice self-compassion and self-love, and to honor your own unique path. Whether you're seeking passion, connection, or simply a deeper understanding of yourself, know that you are worthy of love, pleasure, and fulfillment.

So, as you close this chapter and move forward on your sexual journey, take a moment to celebrate how far you've come, to honor the wisdom you've gained, and to embrace the possibilities that lie ahead. Whether you're experiencing moments of ecstasy or navigating challenges, remember that you are not alone—you have the power to create the fulfilling and satisfying sex life you deserve.